Dash Die

42 Delicioous Dash Diet Recipes For Weight Loss

Sara Banks

Published at Smashwords

Table of Contents

Introduction

I want to thank you and congratulate you for purchasing the book "Dash Diet Recipes-42 Delicious Dash Diet Recipes For Weight Loss"

This book contains proven weight loss ideas and Dash Diet recipes that will help you meet your health and weight loss goals. Research and studies have shown that the Dash Diet reduces the risk of many diseases, including cancer, stroke, heart failure, kidney stones, and diabetes. The Dash Diet was ranked the #1 diet 4 years running by US News and World Report. Come try the diet that thousands of others have already had incredible success with and begin to get healthy and lose weight.

Read it to make your life turn around towards a healthier and fit you!

Thanks again for purchasing this recipe book, I hope you enjoy it!

Sara Banks

What Is the DASH Diet?

It is quite alarming that the number of people suffering from high blood pressure is increasing with each passing day. While high blood pressure may be accelerated by a high salt diet, salt is not the only thing that may cause blood pressure. If you are obese or overweight, you also have a higher chance of having high blood pressure. Other causes of high blood pressure include stress, too much alcohol consumption, old age, genetics and chronic kidney disease as well as other types of adrenal and thyroid disorders.

You may probably be wondering so where does DASH diet come into play. DASH simply stands for Dietary Approaches to Stop Hypertension. This is mainly because the main causes of Hypertension are usually closely related with your diet. Therefore, if you have hypertension, the best way to address the issues is to change your diet rather than rely on pills only. The DASH diet has actually been shown to lower blood pressure within as little as 14 days. Can you imagine this?

What Does the DASH Diet Entail?

This diet plan mainly focuses on consumption of whole grains, nuts, fish, poultry and low fat diet. When on this diet, you consume less of sugar, red meat, fat and sugary drinks. The DASH diet is usually recommended for people with high blood pressure since it meets the low-sodium requirements that are suitable for those suffering from hypertension. Below are some of the nutritional goals of the DASH diet plan:

Fiber is 30 grams

Carbohydrates are 55% calories

Cholesterol is limited to 150 milligrams

Protein is 18% calories

Saturated Fat is 65% calories

Fiber is 30grams

Total Fat is 27% calories

It will also important to know the number of servings of different food groups.

Grains and grain products

These include English muffins, bagels, cereals, grits, whole wheat bread, oatmeal, unsalted pretzels, crackers and popcorn.

The required serving size is 7-8 servings.

An example of such a serving includes: 1 slice of bread, 1 oz dry cereal and ½ cup cooked rice, cereal or pasta.

Since your goal is not to lower blood pressure but to lose weight, you can reduce your carbohydrate intake to 4 to 5 servings.

Vegetables

Vegetables are usually important since they are rich in fiber, magnesium and potassium.

Some common vegetables you can take include potatoes, carrots, green peas, broccoli, squash, spinach, kales, collards, green beans, artichokes, sweet potatoes, lima beans, turnip greens and tomatoes.

The appropriate vegetable serving is 4-5 servings. However, since you have reduced your intake of carbohydrates, you can increase your serving to 5-6 servings.

An example of 4-5 servings include: ½ cup cooked vegetables, 6 ounce vegetable juice and 1 cup raw leafy vegetables.

Fruits

4-5 daily servings of fruits are enough. Some common fruits to take when on a dash diet include grapes, dates, mangoes, tangerines, grapefruit, banana, pineapple, apple, melon, kiwi, avocado, berries and oranges among many other fruits.

A suitable daily serving will be 1 medium fruit, ¼-cup dried fruit, ½-cup fresh fruit and 6 oz. fresh fruit juice.

Low fat or fat free dairy

Dairy products are usually very important, as they are major sources of protein and calcium.

The most appropriate serving when on a dash diet is 2-3 servings.

An example of such a serving is 1 cup yogurt, 8 oz. milk, 1 ½ oz cheese

Meats, Poultry and fish

Meat is an amazing source of magnesium and protein. The recommended serving of meat is 2 or less servings, which is around 3 oz. cooked meat, fish or poultry.

Seeds, Nuts and Dry Beans

Some of these include mixed nuts, walnuts, peanuts, sunflower seeds, lentils, kidney beans, peas and lentils. You are only required to take around 4-5 servings of dry beans, seeds and nuts each week. Nuts can be quite high in salt so try to look for unsalted nuts.

Oils and Fats

2-3 servings of fats and oils daily is just enough. Ensure that you are consuming trans-fat free fats and oils. You do not want to consume more fat and yet you are trying to burn fat. This may however vary depending on the amount of carbohydrates you consume. For instance, if you take fewer carbohydrates, you would want to increase your intake of fats and oils to ensure that your metabolism does not slow down and you still have enough energy.

Suitable serving sizes include 1-teaspoon soft margarine, 1-tablespoon low fat mayonnaise, 1-teaspoon vegetable oil and 2 tablespoons light salad dressing.

Sweets and Sugar

You need to try to keep your intake of things like maple syrup, jelly, sugar, fruit-flavored gelatin, hard candy, ices, fruit punch, sorbet, jellybeans and jam. If you need to take sweets, ensure that they are low in fats.

Dash Diet And Weight Loss

I am sure you are probably wondering 'if the DASH diet is suitable for people who are looking to lower their blood pressure, where do I come in when I want to adopt the diet to lose weight. You will be glad to know that the DASH diet is very relevant if you would want to lose weight. This is mainly because the diet focuses on reduction of intake of sugary foods, processed foods and high carbohydrate foods, which all eventually lead to weight gain. The diet instead focuses on consumption of more fruits, vegetables, healthy fats and more of whole foods.

So how do you lose weight with the DASH Diet? The dash diet enables you to eat more of fruits, vegetables and whole foods that are quite satisfying. What this means is that you will feel hungry less often and thus reducing the number of times you eat throughout the day since you are full. Furthermore, the diet also focuses on consuming a high amount of dairy products that are high in calcium and we all know that calcium rich products favor weight loss. This is mainly since calcium stored in the fat cells usually determines how fat is broken down and stored by the body. This simply means that the more calcium in a fat cell, the more fat it will burn. This is why the meal plan focused greatly on consumption of dairy products. The key is however not to just take any dairy products but rather to take dairy products that are fat-free or low in fat.

Why Does the Dash Diet Work

With there being many diets, you may be wondering which diet to choose. The DASH diet has been shown to be very effective for weight loss due to a number of things even though it was not initially started to achieve weight loss. Most diets usually do not work owing to the high calorie deficit. This is however not the case with this diet. The DASH diet allows you to eat all food groups but in moderation. When you think of all the fad diets that promise fast weight loss, it is usually very hard for you to stick to such a diet. For instance, some people may recommend the consumption of smoothies, juices and a no carb diet in order to lose weight. While you may lose weight, quickly, you are likely to gain it all back again.

DASH diet is not a fad diet but rather a lifestyle diet. Considering that this diet is suitable for people with hypertension, such people need to consume this diet to maintain their blood pressure. You can thus be sure that by adopting this diet, you will not only lose weight but also reduce your risk of getting heart attack, heart failure, stroke and other heart diseases.

Dash Diet Appetizers

1. Grilled Pineapple

Ingredients

1 firm and ripe pineapple

1 tablespoon dark rum

1 tablespoon fresh lime juice

2 tablespoons dark honey

1 tablespoon olive oil

1 tablespoon grated lime zest

¼ teaspoon ground cloves

1 teaspoon ground cinnamon

Instructions

Prepare the grill for high heat.

To make the marinade, combine the olive oil, cinnamon, cloves, limejuice and honey in a large bowl.

Cut the crown of leaves and the base of the pineapple. While keeping the pineapple standing upright, use a large sharp knife to pare off the skin, cutting downward just below the surface in vertical strips. Cut the pineapple, into half lengthwise then place each pineapple half cut side down and cut into four long wedges; remove the core.

Place the pineapple in the bowl with the marinade and stir to coat the pineapple.

Place on the grill and cook for around four minutes, as you baste with the remaining marinade. Turn the fruit and move it to a cooler part of the grill then reduce the heat. Baste again with the marinade and grill until the pineapple is tender and golden brown. This should take around three minutes.

Remove the pineapple from the grill, place on a platter and brush with the rum then sprinkle with the zest. You can serve either warm or hot.

Serves 8.

2. Sweet Chips And Fruit Salsa

Ingredients

For the Fruit Salsa

2 tablespoons orange juice

1 tablespoon honey

3 cups diced fresh fruit like oranges, strawberries, grapes, kiwi or apples

2 tablespoons sugar-free jam

For the tortilla crisps

8 whole-wheat tortillas

½ tablespoon cinnamon

1 tablespoon sugar

Instructions

Preheat the oven to 350F. Cut every tortilla to 10 wedges. Lay the pieces on two baking sheets ensuring that they do not overlap. Spray the pieces with cooking spray.

Combine the cinnamon and sugar in a small bowl. Sprinkle the wedges evenly and bake for 10 to 12 minutes or until crisp. Place them on a cooling rack to cool.

Cut the fruit into cubes then mix them gently in a bowl. Whisk together orange juice and honey in another bowl. Pour this mixture over the diced fruit and mix gently. Cover the bowl with plastic wrap and refrigerate for around two or three hours.

Serve as a topping for the tortilla chips or as a dip.

Serves 10.

3. Fruit Kebabs With Lemon Dip

Ingredients

4 to 6 strawberries

4 to 6 pineapple chunks

4 to 6 grapes

½ banana cut into chunks

1 kiwi, peeled and diced

1 teaspoon lime zest

1 teaspoon fresh lime juice

4 ounces low fat, sugar free lemon yogurt

Instructions

Whisk together the yogurt, lime zest and lime juice. Cover and refrigerate until when needed.

Thread one of each fruit on the skewer. Serve with the lemon lime dip.

Serves 4.

4. Avocado And Pineapple Salsa

Ingredients

1 can of pineapple chunks with pineapple juice

1 avocado, halved, pitted and cubed

1 tablespoon of honey

1 tablespoon fresh lime juice

1 onion, finely chopped

2 tablespoons cilantro leaves, minced

1 jalapeno seeds, removed and diced

1 tablespoon extra virgin olive oil

1 small jalapeno, seeds removed and diced

Salt and Pepper to taste

Instructions

Make the dressing by mixing two tablespoons of pineapple juice with the oil, honey, jalapeno and limejuice. Season with salt and pepper to taste.

Add the onion and pineapple then fold in the cilantro and avocado gently.

Allow the flavors to blend for around 15 minutes before serving.

Serves 6.

5. Garlic Potatoes

Ingredients

1 ¾ lbs potatoes

¾ cup canola oil

2/3 cup all-purpose flour

2 teaspoons chopped parsley

2 cloves of garlic minced

1 teaspoon salt

2 1/3 cups lactose free non-fat milk

Instructions

Preheat the oven to 350 degrees F.

Peel, slice and salt the potatoes. Place some flour in a bowl and dredge the potatoes in the flour.

Heat canola oil in a pan on medium high heat and carefully place a small batch of potatoes in the hot oil and fry until both sides are golden brown.

Remove the potatoes from the pan, place them on a plate lined with paper towels and soak the excess oil.

Let the oil reheat before you can place another batch. Repeat the same process.

Place the fried potatoes in a baking dish and sprinkle with minced garlic. Layer the remaining potatoes on top of the garlic.

Pour the lactose free milk over the potatoes and bake for thirty-five minutes until brown or bubbling. Sprinkle with parsley before serving.

Serves 16.

6. Yogurt Grilled Vegetables

Ingredients

3 zucchini, sliced

2 eggplants, sliced

1 sweet onion

2 cloves garlic, minced

1 ¼ cups plain fat-free yogurt

2 tablespoons olive oil

½ cup balsamic vinegar

½ cup roasted red peppers, diced

2 tablespoons chopped parsley

Instructions

Pour the balsamic vinegar in a pan. Simmer to reduce to three tablespoons then cool the vinegar. Add the vinegar to the oil, yogurt, parsley and garlic mixture. Divide the mixture into half then place the zucchini, onion and eggplant on a sheet pan and brush with ½ of the yogurt mixture.

Cook the vegetables on a lightly oiled preheated grill until golden brown.

Place the vegetables on a platter and sprinkle with red peppers. Drizzle with the remaining dressing and serve.

Serves 4.

Dash Diet Salads

7. Cherry Tomato And Yellow Pear Salad

Ingredients

1 ½ cups halved red cherry tomatoes

1 ½ cups halved orange cherry tomatoes

1 ½ cups yellow pear tomatoes halved

1 tablespoon extra virgin olive oil

1 tablespoon minced shallot

¼ teaspoon salt

4 large basil leaves cut into slender ribbons

2 tablespoons of sherry vinegar

1/8 freshly ground black pepper

Instructions

For the vinaigrette, combine shallot and vinegar and allow it to stand for around 15 minutes. Add the salt, olive oil, and pepper then whisk together until well blended.

Toss together all the tomatoes in a large salad bowl and pour the vinaigrette over the tomatoes then add the basil slender ribbons and toss until well mixed. Serve immediately.

Serves 6.

8. Berry Spinach Salad

Ingredients

1 cup sliced fresh strawberries

4 cups of fresh spinach

1 cup of fresh blueberries

¼ cup chopped toasted pecans

1 sweet onion, sliced

Salad Dressing

2 tablespoons balsamic vinegar

2 tablespoons white wine vinegar

2 teaspoons Dijon mustard

2 tablespoons honey

1/8 teaspoon pepper

1 teaspoon curry powder (optional)

Instructions

Toss together the spinach, blueberries, strawberries, pecans and onions. In a tight fitting jar, combine the dressing ingredients and shake well.

Pour the dressing over the salad and toss to coat. Serve immediately.

Serves 4.

9. Mixed Bean Salad

Ingredients

¼ cup orange juice

1 can (15 ounces) of unsalted black beans, rinsed and drained

¼ cup chopped white onion

1 can (15 ounces) of unsalted green beans, rinsed and drained

½-cup cider vinegar

1 can (15 ounces) of garbanzo beans, rinsed and drained

Sugar substitute (optional)

1 can (15 ounces) of unsalted kidney beans, rinsed and drained

Instructions

Combine the onion and beans in a bowl and mix gently.

Whisk together the vinegar and orange juice in a separate bowl and add the sugar substitute if need be.

Pour the orange juice mixture over the bean mixture. Stir and let it stand for thirty minutes before serving.

Serves 8.

10. Orange Rice Salad

Ingredients

1 can (11 ounces) mandarin oranges with juice

2 cups cooked and cooled brown rice

¾ cup raisins or other dried fruit

2 tablespoons canola oil

¼ cup chopped nuts

½ cup celery, washed and diced

1 tablespoon orange juice

¼ cup parsley chopped

Pepper to taste

Instructions

Mix all ingredients in a medium sized bowl

Chill for around an hour to let the flavors blend.

Refrigerate leftovers within two to three hours.

Serves 7.

11. Carrot Salad With Dried Plums

Ingredients

2 lb carrots, peeled

1 cup pitted dried plums

¼ cup freshly squeezed lemon juice

½ teaspoon hot paprika

2 tablespoons olive oil

¼ teaspoon salt

¼ teaspoon ground cumin

2 tablespoons toasted sesame seeds

3 tablespoons chopped cilantro

Instructions

Cut the carrots into one inch pieces.

Drop carrots in boiling salted water and cook for around five minutes or until tender. Drain and rinse with cold water immediately then put aside.

Whisk together lemon juice, paprika, cumin, cinnamon and salt in a large bowl.

Add in the dried plums, carrots, cilantro, and mix gently.

Serve and sprinkle with sesame seeds.

Serves 6.

12. Broccoli Salad

Ingredients

1 cup raw broccoli, chopped

2 stalks celery, thinly sliced

1 carrot, peeled and diced

½ cup raisins

1 cup cooked ham, chicken or turkey

1 cup plain, non-fat yogurt

¼ cup onion, chopped

¼ cup light mayonnaise

1 teaspoon vinegar

1 tablespoon sugar

Instructions

Mix together the broccoli, celery, carrots, raisins, meat and onion. In a separate bowl, mix together sugar, vinegar and yogurt. Add the mayonnaise mixture to the salad and mix well, then refrigerate the left overs within two to three hours.

Serves 8.

Dash Diet Breakfast Recipes

13. Banana oatmeal pancakes with maple syrup

Ingredients

1 banana, mashed

½ cup rolled oats

½ cup maple syrup

1 cup water

3 whole cloves

½ cinnamon stick

2 tablespoons canola oil

2 tablespoons light brown sugar

½ cup all-purpose flour

½ cup whole wheat flour

¼ teaspoons baking soda

¼ teaspoon ground cinnamon

1 ½ teaspoons baking powder

¼ cup fat-free plain yogurt

½ cup low-fat milk

1 egg, lightly beaten

¼ teaspoon salt

Instructions

Combine the maple syrup, cloves and cinnamon stick in a saucepan. Place the pan over medium heat and bring to a boil. Remove from the heat and allow it to steep for 15 minutes. Remove the cloves and cinnamon stick with a spoon and set the syrup aside then keep warm.

Combine oats and water in a microwave-safe bowl and microwave on high until the oats are tender and creamy. Stir in canola oil and brown sugar and put aside to cool.

Combine the flours, baking soda, baking powder, ground cinnamon and salt. Whisk to ensure it is well blended.

Add milk, banana and yogurt to the oats and stir in until well blended. Beat in the egg, add the flour mixture to the oat mixture, and stir until moistened.

Place a frying pan over medium heat and once hot, spoon ¼ cup batter into the pan. Cook until the top surface is covered with bubbles and the edges lightly browned. Turn and cook until the bottom is well brown. Repeat with the remaining batter.

Place the pancakes on warmed plates, drizzle with warm syrup, and serve.

Serves 6.

14. Egg omelet with Spinach

Ingredients

Cooking Spray

8 eggs

1/8 teaspoon salt

2 tablespoons fresh chives or parsley

1/8 teaspoon cayenne pepper

2 cups fresh baby spinach

½ cup shredded reduced-fat cheddar cheese

Red pepper relish (see recipe below)

Instructions

Coat a non-stick skillet with cooking spray and place over medium heat.

Combine eggs, cayenne pepper, chives, and salt. Whisk until frothy and pour into the skillet. Immediately begin stirring the eggs gently using a wooden spatula until the mixture resembles pieces of cooked eggs that are surrounded by liquid egg. Cook for another thirty seconds until the eggs are set.

Once the egg is set though still shiny, sprinkle with cheese. Top with ¼ cup of the Red pepper relish and 1 cup of baby spinach. Using a spatula, fold one side of the omelet to partially cover the filling. Arrange the remaining spinach on the warm platter. Transfer the omelet to the platter and top with the remaining relish.

Serves 4.

Red Pepper relish

Combine 2 tablespoons finely chopped green onion, 2/3 chopped red sweet pepper, ¼ teaspoon black pepper and 1 tablespoon cider vinegar.

15. Whole Wheat oat Pancakes

Ingredients

½ cup whole-wheat flour

2/3 cup regular oats

1 tablespoon baking powder

½ cup all-purpose flour

¼ teaspoon salt

¼ egg substitute

1 ½ tablespoons vegetable oil

1 cup fat-free milk

¾ cup reduced calorie maple syrup

1 tablespoon powdered sugar

Cooking spray

Instructions

Place oats in a blender and process until ground. Mix the oats, whole-wheat flour, baking powder and all-purpose flour in a bowl. Combine the milk, oil and egg substitute and add to the oats mixture as you stir.

For each pancake, pour ¼ cup batter onto a skillet on high heat coated with cooking spray. Tuck the pancakes once the top is covered with bubbles and the edges look cooked.

Sprinkle the pancakes with the powdered sugar and serve with maple syrup.

Serves 6.

16. Breakfast Fruit Crunch

Ingredients

4 cups assorted fresh fruit like grapefruit, orange, chopped pear, seedless grapes, cubed fresh pineapple and sliced kiwi fruit

2 tablespoons honey

½ cup low fat granola

2 cans (6 ounces each) low fat yogurt

¼-cup coconut toasted

Instructions

Divide the fruit into 6 parfait glasses or bowls

Top the fruit with yoghurt and drizzle with honey.

Sprinkle with coconut and granola.

17. Zucchini lemon muffins

Ingredients

½ cup sugar

2 cups all-purpose flour

2 teaspoons grated lemon rind

1 tablespoon baking powder

½ cup sugar

1 cup shredded zucchini

¼ teaspoon ground nutmeg

¼ teaspoon salt

¾ cup skim milk

Cooking spray

1 egg

3 tablespoons vegetable oil

Instructions

Combine the flour, sugar, baking powder, grated lemon, salt and ground nutmeg in a bowl. Make a well in the center then combine zucchini, oil, milk and egg and stir well. Add to the flour mixture as you stir well until the dry ingredients are well moist.

Divide the batter evenly among the muffin cups and coat with cooking spray. Bake for 20 minutes at 400 degrees. Remove from pans, cool and serve.

18. Apple and Granola Crisp

Ingredients

2 apples

1 tablespoon butter

½ teaspoon grated fresh ginger

Dash of ground cinnamon

4 teaspoons honey

¼ cup low-fat granola

1 tablespoon brown sugar

1 teaspoon lemon zest

1 (6 ounce) fat-free plain yogurt

Instructions

Heat butter in a medium pan over medium heat. Add the apples and cook for around five minutes. Reduce heat to medium-low, stir in brown sugar, cardamom and sugar. Cook and stir for five minutes until the apples are almost tender. Remove from the heat, cover and let stand for ten minutes or until tender.

Combine yoghurt with lemon peel and divide cooked apples among the four bowls. Top with the yoghurt and drizzle with honey and granola.

Serves 4.

19. Broccoli and cheese egg omelets

Ingredients

4 eggs

4 cups of broccoli florets

¼ cup grated parmesan cheese

¼ cup reduced fat cheddar

1 tablespoon olive oil

1 cup egg whites

Cooking spray

Salt and fresh pepper to taste

Instructions

Preheat the oven to 350 degrees F. Steam the broccoli in a little water for around six minutes.

Once the broccoli is cooked, mash into smaller pieces, add olive oil, pepper and salt and mix well.

Spray the muffin tin with cooking spray and spoon the broccoli mixture into the nine tins.

Beat egg whites, parmesan cheese, eggs, salt, pepper and cheese in a bowl. Pour into the greased tins over the broccoli just over ¾ full. Top with the grated cheddar and bake in the oven until cooked. This should take around twenty minutes. Serve immediately.

Serves 9.

20. Fruit And Grain Salad

Ingredients

1 Red apple

1 Granny smith apple

¾ cup brown rice

3 cups water

¾ cup bulgur

1 cup raisins

1 orange

¼ teaspoon salt

1 container (8 oz.) low fat yogurt

Instructions

Heat water in a large pot over high heat.

Add the bulgur and rice and reduce the heat to low. Cover and cook for around ten minutes. Remove from heat and set aside.

Spread the hot grains on the baking sheet to cool.

Prepare the fruits: core and chop the apples and peel the orange and cut into sections.

Transfer the chilled grains and cut fruit into a mixing bowl. Stir in the yoghurt into the grains and fruit until well coated.

Serves 6.

21. Morning Quinoa

Ingredients

1 cup uncooked quinoa

2 cups low fat milk

¼ teaspoon cinnamon

¼ cup honey

¼ cup dried currants

¼ cup sliced almonds

Instructions

Rinse the quinoa thoroughly. Bring milk to boil in a medium pan. Add the quinoa and return to a boil. Cover, reduce the heat to medium low and simmer until almost all the liquid has been absorbed.

Remove from the heat and fluff with a fork. Stir in the remaining ingredients, cover and let it stand for fifteen minutes.

22. Turkey Sausage and Mushroom Strata

Ingredients

12 ounces turkey sausage

8 ounces wheat bread cut into one-inch cubes

1 ½ cup reduced-fat shredded cheddar cheese

½ teaspoon paprika

3 large eggs

2 cups fat free milk

1 cup sliced mushrooms

12 ounces egg substitute

2 tablespoons grated parmesan cheese

Black pepper to taste

Instructions

Preheat oven to 400 degrees F.

Arrange the bread cubes on a baking sheet and bake for 8 minutes or until toasted.

Heat a pan over medium heat. Add sausage and cook for seven minutes until it starts to crumble. Combine the eggs, cheese, egg substitute, paprika, salt, parmesan cheese and pepper in a bowl. Cover and refrigerate for eight hours or through the night.

Preheat the oven to 350 degrees. Uncover the casserole and bake for 50 minutes at 350 degrees F. Cut into twelve pieces and serve.

Serves 12.

Dash Diet Main Dishes

23. Roasted Turkey

Ingredients

1 whole turkey, thawed

4 garlic cloves, finely chopped

1 medium shallot, peeled and chopped finely

2 carrots, finely chopped

Coarse black pepper to taste

8 Roma tomatoes cut in half through the stem

2 yellow onions chopped

2 celery stalks, chopped

Instructions

Preheat the oven to 400F.

Add the shallots, black pepper and garlic in a small bowl and mix properly then put aside.

Arrange the onion, celery and carrots in the bottom of a roasting pan. Unwrap your turkey from the packaging and discard fatty tissues, giblets and neck. Rinse the turkey inside out and pat dry using paper towels.

Put the turkey breast-side up on top of the vegetables in your roasting pan and tuck the wing tips behind the turkey's back. Rub the turkey with the shallot mixture and arrange the tomatoes around the outside of the turkey. Place in the middle part of the oven and cook uncovered.

Bake at 400F for twenty minutes then reduce the temperature to 325F. Check the doneness after the bird has roasted for around three hours. You will know if the bird is done if you pierce and juices run clear.

As the turkey is in the oven, put the turkey neck in a small pan, add four cups of water and place over medium heat. Cover and simmer for at least one hour. You can use the stock for your gravy or freeze it to use it as a base for some soup.

Remove the turkey from the roasting pan and put on a platter. Remove the vegetables using a slotted spoon and arrange around the turkey. Cover the vegetables and turkey with aluminum foil and let it rest for twenty minutes before you can carve.

Carve and serve.

24. Citrus Chicken

Ingredients

3 skinned and boned chicken breasts cut into two inch pieces

1 ½ cups orange juice

2 teaspoons vegetable oil

1 clove garlic minced

½ teaspoon minced ginger

1 can (8 ounce) pineapple chunks, drained (keep the juice)

1 cup water or reduced-sodium chicken broth

4 cups sliced vegetables like green peppers, mushrooms, onions and celery

2 tablespoons cornstarch

1 tablespoon sugar

2 tablespoons vinegar

1 tomato, cut in wedges

2 tablespoons reduced-sodium soy sauce

Instructions

Heat oil in a large pan over medium heat. Once hot, add the ginger, garlic and chicken and cook for around five minutes until the chicken is not pink.

Add 1 cup of orange juice, pineapple juice, vinegar and chicken broth. Cover and simmer for five minutes.

Add the sliced vegetables and cook for around three minutes.

Mix the remaining ½ cup of orange juice with soy sauce, cornstarch and sugar in a bowl. Stir until smooth then add to the skillet and cook while stirring consistently until the mixture boils and starts to thicken.

Add the pineapple chunks and tomato wedges. Serve.

Serves 10.

25. Mustard Glazed Ribs

Ingredients

3 lb pork ribs cut into individual ribs

1 cup ketchup

3 tablespoons brown mustard

1/3 cup cider vinegar

2 tablespoons brown sugar

1 teaspoon onion powder

¼ teaspoon hot sauce

1 onion, diced

3 tablespoons water

Instructions

Heat the oven to 400 degrees F. Place, the ribs in a baking dish and cover tightly with foil. Bake for one hour and drain off any accumulated liquid.

In a medium-size pan, stir together the vinegar, ketchup, brown sugar, mustard, water, hot sauce and the onion powder. Cook for ten minutes over medium heat as you stir continuously. Place half the sauce in a bowl and put aside.

Heat the grill to medium high, then coat the grill rack lightly with oil or nonstick cooking spray.

Baste the ribs with the remaining sauce and grill for three minutes each side. Serve the ribs with the reserved sauce.

Serves 6.

26. Pear Chicken Curry

Ingredients

3 boneless, skinless chicken breasts, halved and cut into one inch cubes

2 ripe pears, divided

1 cup diced onion

1 tablespoon vegetable oil

1 teaspoon minced garlic

1 tablespoon curry powder

1 teaspoon salt

¾ teaspoon ground cinnamon

¾ teaspoon ground ginger

¼ teaspoon ground black pepper

1/3 cup raisins (optional)

1 can (14 ounces) coconut milk

Instructions

Peel and core the one pear, puree and put aside.

Heat the oil in a large pan over medium heat. Add the onion, garlic, curry powder, ginger, salt, pepper, cinnamon and salt and sauté for five minutes or until the onions are transparent.

Add the chicken and sauté for five minutes as you stir frequently until browned. Add the pureed pear, coconut milk and raisins. Simmer for five minutes. Core and cut the other pear into ½-inch cubes and add to the curry. Simmer for five minutes then serve.

Serves 6.

27. Lime Tilapia Tacos

Ingredients

1 lb tilapia fillets, rinsed and dry

3 tablespoons lime juice

1 onion, chopped

1 teaspoon olive oil

2 jalapeno peppers, chopped

4 cloves garlic minced

2 cups diced tomatoes

¼ cup fresh cilantro chopped

Salt and pepper to taste

8 5-inch tortillas

1 cup shredded cabbage

1 medium avocado, sliced

Fresh cilantro and lime wedges to garnish

4 tablespoons low-fat sour cream (optional)

Instructions

Heat oil in a pan and sauté the onion until translucent then add garlic and mix well.

Place the tilapia in the pan and cook until the flesh starts to flake.

Add the jalapeno peppers, cilantro, lime juice and tomatoes

Sauté over medium heat for around five minutes, as you break the fish up to mix everything well.

Season with salt and pepper to taste.

Meanwhile, heat the tortillas on a pan for a few minutes until each side is warm.

Serve a little over ¼ cup of fish on each warmed tortilla with two avocado slices.

Split a ¼ cup of the shredded cabbage and 1 tablespoon of the low fat sour cream between two tacos.

Garnish with lime wedges and fresh chopped cilantro.

Serves 4.

28. Ginger Chicken with Rice Noodles

Ingredients

2 skinless, boneless halved chicken breasts

1 ½ teaspoons grated ginger

2 ounces dried rice noodles

2 tablespoons finely chopped green onion

1/8 teaspoon salt

3 cloves garlic, minced

3 teaspoons olive oil

½ teaspoon finely shredded lime peel

½ cup chopped carrot

1 tablespoon fresh cilantro

2 tablespoons chopped peanuts

1 teaspoon lime juice

1 teaspoon chopped green onion

Instructions

Combine the green onion, garlic, ginger, salt and one teaspoon of oil and sprinkle over the chicken.

Place the chicken on the rack of an uncovered grill and grill for 12 to 15 minutes or until tender.

Meanwhile, cook rice noodles and carrot in a large saucepan of boiling water until the noodles are tender. Rinse with cold water and drain again. You can snip the noodles into short lengths using a kitchen scissors.

Stir together lime peel, two teaspoons of oil and lime juice. Add the noodle mixture and cilantro and mix.

Divide the noodles into two individual bowls and arrange the chicken slices on the noodle mixture. Sprinkle with peanuts and serve.

Serves 2.

29. Swordfish tacos with cilantro and lime

Ingredients

1 ¾ lbs swordfish fillets or steaks

2 tomatoes, seeded and diced

¾ cup pitted black olives, chopped

½ jalapeno chili, seeded and minced

3 green onions, sliced

1 teaspoon grated lime zest

4 tablespoons fresh lime juice

3 tablespoons extra-virgin olive oil

1 tablespoon rice vinegar

½ teaspoon salt

4 tablespoons chopped fresh cilantro

¼ teaspoon pepper

1 cup grated radishes

1 head romaine lettuce, sliced thinly

1 teaspoon chili powder

½ roasted and seeded red bell pepper

12 corn tortillas

1 teaspoon ground cumin

Instructions

Combine the diced tomatoes, olives, jalapeno, green onions, lime zest, two tablespoons of lime juice, two tablespoons of cilantro, two tablespoons of olive oil, salt and pepper. Toss gently until all the ingredients have been distributed evenly. Cover and refrigerate. Place the radishes and romaine in separate bowls, cover and refrigerate.

Cut the roasted bell pepper into chunks. Combine the roasted pepper, ¼ teaspoon chili powder, ½ cup chopped tomatoes, 2 tablespoons lime juice and ¼ teaspoon cumin and pulse. Stir in the remaining two tablespoons of cilantro then put aside.

Preheat the oven to 300F, wrap the tortillas in aluminum foil, and warm in the oven for around ten minutes. Remove from the oven and keep warm.

Raise the oven temperature to 400F. Toss the swordfish cubes with the remaining olive oil, cumin and chili powder and arrange the fish in a single layer on the baking sheet. Bake the fish until it is opaque. This should take around five minutes

When serving, place two tortillas on each plate, divide the tomato olive mixture into two, and top with equal portions of fish. Add the radishes and lettuce to each and drizzle with lime-cilantro.

Serves 6.

30. Pasta with grilled chicken, mushrooms and white beans

Ingredients

2 boneless, skinless chicken breasts

1 cup cooked white beans

1 cup sliced mushrooms

1 tablespoon olive oil

2 tablespoons chopped garlic

½ cup chopped white onion

¼ cup chopped fresh basil

¼ cup Parmesan cheese

12 ounces uncooked pasta

Ground black pepper to taste

Instructions

Preheat the grill for high heat. Coat the grill rack lightly with cooking oil and position it four inches from the heat source.

Broil the chicken until brown and just cooked. This should take around five minutes each side. Cut the chicken into strips once cooled for five minutes

Heat olive oil in a large frying pan over medium heat. Add the mushrooms, onions, and sauté until tender. This should take around five minutes. Stir in the garlic, white beans, grilled chicken strips and basil.

Fill a large pot with water and bring to boil. Add the pasta and cook for around ten minutes or depending on the directions on the package. Drain the pasta thoroughly.

Return the pasta to the pot, add the chicken mixture and toss to mix evenly. Divide the pasta between the plates and garnish with one tablespoon of parmesan cheese and black pepper to taste. Serve immediately.

Serves 4.

31. Mango Salsa Pizza

Ingredients

½ cup mango, seeded, peeled and chopped

½ cup minced onion

½ cup pineapple tidbits

½ cup fresh cilantro, chopped

1 tablespoon lime juice

1 ½ inch whole grain prepared pizza crust

Instructions

Preheat the oven to 425 F. Coat lightly a baking pan with cooking spray.

Combine the onions, peppers, pineapple, mango, cilantro and lime juice and put aside.

Roll out the dough and press into the baking pan. Cook in the oven for around fifteen minutes.

Take the pizza crust out and spread with the mango salsa. Place the pizza back into the oven and bake until the toppings are hot and the crust has browned. This should take around five to ten minutes.

Cut the pizza into 8 even slices.

Serve immediately. Serves 4.

32. White Beans with Spinach, Shrimp and Feta

Ingredients

1 can (15 ounces) unsalted cannellini beans, rinsed and drained

5 cups baby spinach

1 lb shrimp, peeled and deveined

2 tablespoons balsamic vinegar

2 tablespoons olive oil

4 cloves garlic, minced

1 medium onion, chopped

2 teaspoons of chopped fresh sage

1 ½ cup low sodium, fat-free feta cheese

Instructions

Heat one teaspoon of oil in a large non-stick pan over medium-high heat. Cook the shrimp until it is opaque. This should take around three minutes. Once cooked, transfer to a plate.

Heat the remaining oil in the same pan over medium heat and add onion, sage and garlic and cook for four minutes as you stir occasionally until golden. Add in the vinegar and cook for thirty seconds.

Add the broth, bring to boil and cook for two minutes. Stir in the spinach and beans and cook until the spinach wilts; this should take around two to three minutes.

Remove from the heat and stir in the shrimp. Top with feta cheese.

Serves 4.

Dash Diet Desserts

33. Yogurt With Fresh Strawberries And Honey

Ingredients

3 cups plain low-fat yogurt

4 tablespoons toasted sliced almonds

4 teaspoons honey

1 pint fresh strawberries

Instructions

Clean and slice the strawberries into quarters then set aside

Place ¾ cup of the yogurt into four serving dishes. Divide the strawberries evenly among the dishes. Top each with a teaspoon of honey then a teaspoon of toasted almonds.

Serve immediately. Serves 4.

34. Milk Chocolate Pudding

Ingredients

2 tablespoons cocoa powder

3 tablespoons cornstarch

1/8 teaspoon salt

2 tablespoons sugar

2 cups non-fat milk

½ teaspoon vanilla

1/3 cup chocolate chips

Instructions

Mix the cornstarch, sugar, cocoa powder and sugar in a saucepan until well mixed then add in milk and whisk. Heat over medium heat as you continue stirring frequently until it thickens. Remove from heat and stir in vanilla and the chocolate chips until melted and smooth.

Pour into a large dish and chill. Place plastic wrap over the surface to prevent a skin from forming on top.

Serves 4.

35. Mixed Berry Pie

Ingredients

¾ cup raspberries

12 strawberries, sliced

½ cup fat free, sugar free instant vanilla pudding made using low-fat or fat-free milk

6 tablespoons light whipped topping

6 single serve graham cracker pie crusts

6 mint leaves for garnishing

Instructions

Mix the raspberries and strawberries in a small bowl.

Spoon 4 teaspoons of the pudding into every pie crust. Add the two tablespoons of the raspberry-strawberry mixture into each pie. Top with one tablespoon of whipped topping and garnish with mint leaves.

Serve immediately.

Serves 6.

36. Grapes and walnuts with sour cream

Ingredients

1 ½ cups red seedless grapes

3 tablespoons chopped walnuts

½ cup fat-free sour cream

2 tablespoons powdered sugar

½ teaspoon lemon juice

½ teaspoon lemon zest

1/8 teaspoon vanilla extract

Instructions

Combine sour cream, lemon zest, powdered sugar, vanilla and lemon juice. Whisk, then cover and chill for several hours.

Divide the grapes among 6 dessert bowls then add two tablespoons of the lemon topping on every dish and sprinkle each bowl with ½ tablespoon of chopped walnuts.

Serve immediately. Serves 6.

37. Chocolate Pie

Ingredients

4 oz. white chocolate, finely chopped

¼ cup sugar

½ lb cream cheese

½ cup heavy cream, chilled

1/3 cup sour cream

1 banana, sliced

1 readymade graham cracker crust around 9 inches.

1 teaspoon vanilla extract

Instructions

Warm the chocolate in a bowl over a pot of simmering water. When partially melted, remove from the heat and stir to melt completely.

Beat the sugar, vanilla and cream cheese until smooth. Beat in the sour cream and chocolate.

Whip the heavy cream until firm then gently fold into the chocolate filling.

Put the banana slices on the crust and top with the filling then chill for two hours. You can sprinkle with dark chocolate before serving.

38. Berry Banana Ice cream

Ingredients

1 cup frozen berries

3 bananas cut into one inch pieces and frozen

1 ½ teaspoons vanilla extract

½ cup non-fat milk

Instructions

Put the frozen bananas in a food processor, add milk and vanilla and process for one minute. Once a smooth consistency has been achieved, add the berries and pulse until they are in pieces and incorporated into the banana mixture.

Serve immediately.

Serves 4.

Dash Diet Soups

39. Potato Soup with apples and cheese

Ingredients

6 potatoes, peeled and sliced

4 large granny apples, cored and peeled and quartered

One Granny smith apple, cored and sliced thinly for garnishing

1 cup chopped yellow onion

2 cups low-sodium chicken broth

¼ cup sliced leeks

¼ teaspoon dried thyme

4 ounces brie cheese, cut into cubes

3 cups fat-free evaporated milk

Instructions

Spray a soup pot with some cooking spray. Add the leeks, onion and four of the apples. Sauté over medium heat until well softened. Add the chicken broth, thyme and bay leaf and bring to a boil. Reduce the heat to low and simmer for around fifteen minutes. Turn off the heat, remove the bay leaf and set aside.

As the broth mixture is cooking, combine the evaporated milk and potatoes in a separate pan. Cook over medium heat until the potatoes are tender. Stir frequently; pour the potato mixture into the soup pot, and mix evenly.

Puree the soup in batches in a blender and puree until smooth. Add the pieces of brie cheese as you puree. Return the pureed batch to the soup pot and heat until warm. Serve in individual bowls and garnish with thin slices of apple.

Serve immediately. Serves 8.

40. Roasted butternut squash soup

Ingredients

1 butternut squash

1 cup diced celery

2 teaspoons canola oil

1 ½ cup spinach

1 cup diced carrot

2 cloves garlic, minced

1 teaspoon sage

4 cups unsalted vegetable stock

1 ½ cups of diced yellow onion

1 teaspoon black pepper

½ teaspoon nutmeg

Instructions

Cut the squash into ½ -inch pieces, put in a roasting pan and add teaspoon of oil. Roast at 400 F for forty minutes or until brown.

Add the remaining oil to a large pot. Add in the vegetables and sauté over medium-high heat or until the vegetables are browned light. Add the spices, squash and stock to the pot and simmer for a few minutes.

Puree the soup carefully with a stick blender. Process the soup in batches and return the pureed soup to the pot then let it simmer. Serve

Serves 4.

41. Shamrock soup

Ingredients

¾ cup dry split peas, rinsed and drained

½ cup chopped onion

½ cup chopped celery

½ cup chopped carrot

1 tablespoon butter

1 ½ cups fat free milk, divided

4 tablespoons diced and fully cooked lean ham

Ground black pepper to taste

4 cups washed and dried fresh spinach leaves

1 can (13 ounces) chicken broth

Pinch of ground nutmeg

Instructions

Sauté onion, celery and carrot in butter in a medium pan until soft. Add the peas, half the milk and the chicken broth. Bring to boil and reduce the heat to low and simmer for thirty minutes while stirring occasionally until the split peas are tender.

Remove from the heat and allow to cool. Puree split pea mixture with spinach in a blender and return the mixture to the saucepan. Add in the remaining milk and stir to achieve the desired consistency.

Cook and stir over low heat until the mixture starts to simmer. Season to taste with ground pepper and nutmeg. Ladle into bowls and sprinkle with ham.

Serves 4.

42. Creamy mushroom Soup

Ingredients

1 ½ lbs sliced white mushrooms

2 teaspoons butter

½ cup thinly sliced green onions

1 cup diced carrots

1 teaspoon minced garlic

¼ teaspoon ground black pepper

1 cup white wine

¼ teaspoon dried thyme

1 ½ cups low-fat milk

1 can (14 ounces) low sodium vegetable broth

¼ teaspoon ground black pepper

Instructions

Melt butter in a large pan over medium heat. Add the onions, carrots, garlic, pepper and thyme and cook as you stir frequently until the onions just start to brown; this should take around five minutes.

Add the wine, mushroom and broth and bring to boil. Cook for one minute and then using a slotted spoon, remove one cup of the vegetables and put aside.

Puree half of the remaining soup from the pan and put in a bowl. Repeat with the remaining mixture until you have pureed the entire soup from the pan. Stir in the milk and the vegetables you had set aside. Simmer until it has just heated through. This should take around five minutes.

Garnish with the sliced green onions if your desire.

Serves 8.

7-Day Meal Plan

Day One

Breakfast

Herbal Tea

1 cup low-fat milk

1 bran muffin

1 teaspoon trans-fat free margarine

¼ cup fresh mixed fruits like banana, apple, berries and melons

Snack

Tail mix made with ¼ cup raisins

Lunch

Chicken curry wrap made with:

1 medium whole-wheat tortilla

½ cup chopped apple

3 ounces chopped and cooked chicken

2 tablespoons fat-free mayonnaise

8 raw baby carrots

Afternoon Snack

A slice of pineapple

Dinner

1 cup cooked whole-wheat spaghetti with a cup of marinara sauce

2 cups mixed salad greens

1 tablespoon low-fat Caesar dressing

1 teaspoon trans-free margarine

½ cup low fat milk

1 nectarine

Day two

Breakfast

1 cup fat-free milk

1 whole-wheat bagel

2 tablespoons peanut butter

1 small banana

Snack

1 cup fat-free yoghurt

Lunch

1 Cup fat-free milk

Turkey Sandwich

½ cup baby carrots

1 medium apple

Dinner

1 cup brown rice pilaf

Baked Chicken Breast

½ cup green beans

1 cup salad

A cup of berries

Day Three

Day 1

Breakfast

6 ounces tomato juice

2 slices of bacon

Hardboiled Egg

Snack

Baby Carrots

1 slice of light cheese

Lunch

Swordfish tacos with cilantro and lime

Cherry tomatoes

1 cup Sugar-Free Strawberry Jell-O

Snack

12 cashews

Dinner

Pasta with grilled chicken, mushrooms and white beans

1 cup of fat-free milk

1 cup mixed fruit

Day Four

Breakfast

1 cup fat-free milk

1 small whole-wheat bagel with one tablespoon peanut butter

1 orange

Snack

1 cup fat-free yogurt

Lunch

Spinach salad made with:

3 cups fresh spinach

1 sliced pear

¼ cup canned mandarin orange sections

2 tablespoons reduced-fat red wine vinaigrette

1/3 cup silvered almonds

½ cup fat-free milk

Snack

2 Vanilla wafers

Dinner

½ cup brown rice pilaf

2 ounces herb-crusted baked Cod

½ cup steamed green beans

1 teaspoon trans-fat free margarine

1 cup chopped berries with mint

Day Five

Breakfast

Broccoli and Cheese Egg omelet

1 cup low-fat milk

1 Banana

Snack

1 Apple

Lunch

2 Turkey Swiss roll-ups

½ cup coleslaw

1 cup snow peas

1 cup of mixed fruit

Snack

¼ cup toasted walnuts

Dinner

Roasted Sliced Turkey

Sautéed onions and carrots

Side Salad with low-fat dressing

Banana Berry Ice cream

Day Six

Breakfast

2 Scrambled eggs

2 slices of bacon

4 ounces cranberry juice

Snack

1 cup of Low-fat vanilla yoghurt

Lunch

Coconut Fried Chicken Breast

1 cup of coleslaw

1 cup Baby carrots

1 banana

Snack

Grapes and Walnuts with Sour Cream

Dinner

Turkey and vegetable Stir fry

1 cup broccoli

Salad with balsamic dressing

Grilled pineapple

Day Seven

Breakfast

1 cup fat-free milk

1 slice whole-wheat toast

1 Scrambled egg

1 tablespoon jam

1 Apple

Snack

10 almonds

Lunch

2 Muester cheese and roast beef roll-ups

Coleslaw

1 peach

Snack

1 cup fat-free strawberry yogurt

Dinner

Avocado and pineapple salsa

Mustard glazed ribs

A small slice of chocolate pie

Conclusion

It is such a pity that we are an overweight society that is always eating processed foods and foods that are high in sugars. It's no wonder that we are seeing very high numbers of people who are obese or overweight. If you need to lose weight, you need to take the right steps to achieve this. Adopting the DASH diet is a great idea considering all the benefits of this diet like not having to starve yourself in order to lose weight. With this diet, you are sure that you will not only lose weight but will also adopt better eating habits that will enable you to live a healthier life.

I hope this book will enable you to make healthier choices to enable you achieve your desired weight loss goals.

Thank you again for purchasing this book!

Sara Banks

CPSIA information can be obtained at www.ICGtesting.com
Printed in the USA
BVOW02s0859240116

434042BV00040B/2003/P